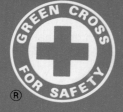

National Safety Council

First Aid and CPR

Second Edition

Level 1

The first aid and CPR procedures in this book are based on the most current recommendations of responsible medical sources. The National Safety Council and the publisher, however, make no guarantee as to, and assume no responsibility for, the correctness, sufficiency or completeness of such information or recommendations. Other or additional safety measures may be required under particular circumstances.

Library of Congress Cataloging-in-Publication Data

First aid and CPR. Level 1/National Safety Council—2nd ed.
   p. cm.
  Includes bibliographical references and index.
  ISBN 0-86720-792-2
  1. First aid in illness and injury. 2. CPR (First aid) I. National SafetyCouncil.
  RC86.7.F558   1993
  616.02'52—dc20   93-221430
                                           CIP

Vice President and Publisher ■ Clayton E. Jones

Director of Production ■ Paula Carroll
Design and Production ■ PC&F, Inc.
Cover Design ■ Hannus Design Associates

Principal Photographer ■ Rick Nye
Illustrations ■ Chris Young, artist
Greg Kyle, Larry Hall, Matt Hall, illustrators
Other full-color illustrations ■
  Bruce Argyle, M.D.
  H.B. Bectal, M.D.
  Michael D. Ellis
  Murray P. Hamlet, D.V.M.
  Axel W. Hoke, M.D.
  Sherman A. Minton, M.D.
  Eugene Robertson, M.D.
  Richard C. Ruffalo, D.M.D.
  Jeffrey Saffle, M.D.
  Clifford C. Snyder, M.D.
  Charles E. Stewart, M.D.
  Health Edco

Jones and Bartlett Publishers
40 Tall Pine Drive
Sudbury, MA 01776
(508) 443-5000

Printed in the United States of America
10 9 8

Welcome Message

Congratulations on your decision to take National Safety Council first aid training. More than 140,000 Americans die every year from injuries, and one in three suffers a nonfatal injury, so it is likely that at some time in your life you will encounter an emergency requiring first aid.

Your training in what to do and how to do it may help keep someone alive or prevent a more serious injury. Emergencies can happen anywhere and at any time.

We hope you will enjoy learning more about first aid through the careful study and application of the concepts being taught. Your training can make it possible for you to act confidently if someone needs help when seconds count.

It is wonderful to be able to save a life or aid someone who has been injured! Protecting life and promoting health have been the Council's only mission since 1913.

On behalf of the National Safety Council, as well as our local safety councils and training agencies, I wish you success in your first aid training program.

Sincerely,

Gerard F. Scannell

Gerard F. Scannell, President
National Safety Council

Table of Contents

1

Introduction

The Size of the Injury Problem

Injuries are one of the most serious public health problems. Injuries are the leading cause of death and disability in children and young adults. They destroy the health, lives, and livelihoods of millions of people.

- Each year, more than 140,000 Americans die from injuries (including accidents, suicides, and homicides), and one person in three suffers a nonfatal injury.
- Preceded by heart disease, cancer, and stroke, injury is the fourth leading cause of death among all Americans.
- One of every eight hospital beds is occupied by an injured patient.
- Every year, more than 80,000 Americans

Percentages of years of potential life lost to injury, cancer, heart disease, and other diseases before age 65. Modified from Centers for Disease Control.

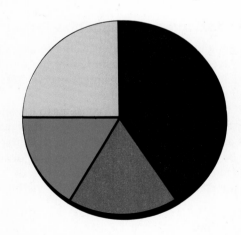

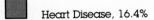 Heart Disease, 16.4%

Cancers, 18.0%

Injury, 40.8%

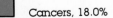 All other diseases, 24.8%

suffer unnecessary but permanently disabling injuries of the brain or spinal cord.
- Injury is the leading reason for physician contacts. And more than 25% of hospital emergency room visits are for the treatment of injuries.

Need for First Aid Training

Because of the size and magnitude of the injury problem, everyone must expect sooner or later to be present when an injury or sudden illness strikes. The outcome of such misfortune frequently depends not only on the severity of the injury or illness, but on the first aid rendered. Therefore, every person should be trained in first aid.

First aid is the immediate care given to the injured or suddenly ill person. First aid does *not* take the place of proper medical treatment. It consists only of furnishing temporary assistance until competent medical care, *if needed*, is obtained, or until the chance for recovery without medical care is assured. **Most injuries and illnesses require only first aid care**.

Properly applied, first aid may mean the difference between life and death, rapid recovery and long hospitalization, or temporary disability and permanent injury.

Legal Aspects of First Aid

Duty to Act

No one is required to render aid when no legal duty to do so exists. For example, even a physician could ignore a stranger suffering a heart attack or a fractured bone. Moral obligations exist, but they may not be the same as a legal obligation to give aid.

Duty to act may occur in the following situations:

1. **When employment requires it.** If your employment has designated you to render first aid and you are called to an accident scene, then you have a duty to act. Examples include law enforcement officers, park rangers, lifeguards, and teachers who have a job description usually designating the giving of first aid.

2. *When a preexisting responsibility exists.* You may have a preexisting relationship with another person which demands being responsible for them (e.g., parent-child, driver-passenger) although it is not spelled out in your job description. You must give first aid should they need it.

3. *After beginning first aid.* Once you start first aid, you cannot stop. Duty to give first aid is usually questioned only when a person fails to act.

Standards of Care

Standards of care ensure quality care and protection for injured or suddenly sick victims. The elements making up a standard of care include:

1. *The type of rescuer.* A first aider should provide the level and type of care expected of a reasonable person with the same amount of training and in similar circumstances.

2. *Published recommendations.* Emergency care-related organizations and societies publish recommended first aid procedures. For example, the American Heart Association publishes procedures for giving CPR.

Obtain Consent to Help

You should obtain the victim's approval or permission before starting first aid. This permission is known as **consent.**

- When a victim gives permission to a first aider to help, this is known as **actual consent.** Oral or written permission is valid.
- Consent should be obtained from every conscious, mentally competent adult.
- Permission is implied for giving care for an unconscious victim and is known as **implied consent.** A first aider should not hesitate to treat an unconscious victim.
- Consent should be obtained from the parent or guardian of a victim who is a child, or of one who is an adult but is mentally incompetent. If a parent or guardian is not available, emergency first aid to maintain life may be given without consent. Do *not* withhold first aid from a minor just to obtain parental or guardian permission.
- Psychological emergencies present difficult problems of consent. Under most conditions, a police officer is the only person with the authority to restrain and transport a person against the person's will. However, if the victim is not violent, the situation is similar to that for minors.

Abandonment

Abandonment refers to the behavior of a first aider who begins giving care and then leaves the victim before another person arrives to take over. After starting first aid, you must remain with the victim until he or she is under the care of another person with equal or more training, or until the victim refuses treatment or transportation.

The Right to Refuse Care

A difficult problem involves the conscious, rational, adult victim who is suffering from an actual or potential life-threatening injury or illness but who refuses treatment or transportation. In such situations, make every reasonable effort to convince the victim, or anyone who can influence the victim, to accept first aid and/or transportation. When such a victim refuses to consent, do *not* give first aid or transportation. In such cases, document everything on paper, and if possible, have witnesses.

Parent Refusing Permission to Help a Child

Very rarely will a first aider encounter a parent who refuses permission—usually on moral, ethical, or religious grounds—to care for a seriously injured or ill child. If refusal does occur, make every effort to convince the parent about the seriousness of the problem and the necessity of first aid. If you do not succeed, call the police, document everything on paper, and if possible, have witnesses.

The Intoxicated or Belligerent Victim

If an intoxicated or belligerent victim refuses first aid, make every effort to persuade him or her of the need for such care. If refused, document everything in writing; if possible, have witnesses.

If the intoxicated person consents to first aid, take the greatest possible care. Alcohol and drugs may hide signs and symptoms of an injury. Because first aiders may be repulsed by the appearance and/or attitude of the intoxicated person, they may overlook injuries. It's important to focus on helping the victim.

Good Samaritan Laws

First aiders are covered by a Good Samaritan law in some states. The Good Samaritan laws protect only those acting in good faith and without gross negligence or willful misconduct. If first aiders provide care within the scope of their training, lawsuits are rare. However, if a minor injury is worsened by a first aider, litigation is possible.

2

Victim Assessment

Do *not* move the injured or suddenly ill person until you have a clear idea of the injury or illness and have applied first aid. The exception occurs when the victim is exposed to further danger at the accident scene. If the injury is serious, if it occurred in an area where the victim can remain safely, and if emergency medical service (EMS) attention is readily available, it is sometimes best not to attempt to move the person, but to use first aid at the injury scene until the EMS system responds.

When making a victim assessment, a first aider will consider what witnesses to the accident can tell about the accident, what is observed about the victim, and what the victim can tell.

The first aider must not assume that the obvious injuries are the only ones present because less noticeable injuries may also have occurred. Look for the causes of the injury which may provide a clue as to the extent of physical damage.

In all actions taken during the initial survey the first aider should be especially careful not to move the victim any more than necessary to support life. Any unnecessary movement or rough handling should be avoided because it might aggravate undetected fractures or spinal injuries.

In order to provide good first aid, a person should be able to identify a victim's injury or sudden illness and determine its seriousness. To find out what is wrong and how extensive it is, the first aider should follow a systematic approach known as a victim assessment. Often an abbreviated assessment is sufficient.

A victim assessment attempts to:

- Gain the victim's consent
- Gain the victim's confidence
- Identify the victim's problems and determine which of them require immediate first aid
- Get information about the victim that may prove useful later to the EMS responders and attending medical personnel

A victim assessment of either an injured victim or a medically ill victim is divided into two steps:

- Primary survey
- Secondary survey

Primary Survey

The primary survey covers these areas:

    A—Airway open?
    B—Breathing?
    C—Circulation at carotid pulse?
    H—Hemorrhage: severe bleeding?

The primary survey is the first step in assessing a victim. Its purpose is to find and correct life-threatening conditions.

Airway. Ask: Does the victim have an open airway? If the person is talking or is conscious, the airway is open. Refer to page 8 for the correct and detailed procedures.

Breathing. Ask: Is the victim breathing? Conscious victims are breathing. However, note any breathing difficulties or unusual breathing sounds. If the victim is unconscious, keep the airway open and *look* for the chest to rise and fall, *listen* for breathing, and *feel* for air coming out of the victim's nose and mouth. See page 9 for the correct and detailed procedures.

Circulation. Ask: Is the victim's heart beating? Determine this by feeling for a pulse at the side of the neck (carotid pulse). Refer to page 10 for the correct and detailed procedures.

Hemorrhage. Ask: Is the victim severely bleeding? Check for severe bleeding by looking, if necessary, over the victim's entire body for blood-soaked clothing as a sign of severe bleeding. See Chapter 5 for the correct and detailed procedures.

Secondary Survey

Having completed the primary survey and attended to any life-threatening problems it uncovers, take a closer look at the victim and make a systematic assessment called the secondary survey.

Look for important signs and symptoms of injury. A **sign** is something the first aider sees, hears, or feels (e.g., pale face, no respiration, cool skin). A **symptom** is something the victim tells the first aider about (e.g., nausea, back pain, no sensation in the extremities).

TABLE 2–4 Victim Assessment

Scene Survey

- dangerous hazards?   - number of victims?   - cause of injury?

Primary Survey (also known as Basic Life Support (BLS))

Check responsiveness/protect spine

A = Airway open? (head-tilt/chin-lift)
B = Breathing? (look at chest; listen and feel for air)
C = Circulation? (pulse at carotid?)
H = Hemorrhage? (severe bleeding; personal protection)

Secondary Survey

Interview

- Introduce self/reassure/victim's name/obtain consent/ask questions:

S = Signs/Symptoms (chief complaint)?
   P = Period of pain (how long)?
   A = Area (where)?
   I = Intensity?
   N = Nullify (what stops it)?
A = Allergies?
M = Medications currently taking?
P = Pertinent past medical history?
L = Last oral intake: solid or liquid? when and how much?
E = Events leading to injury or illness?

Vital signs

- Pulse: rate?
- Respiration: rate/sounds?
- Skin condition: temperature/color/moisture?
- Capillary refill?

Head-to-Toe Examination (use LAF: L = Look; A = Ask; F = Feel)

Head:	- Bleeding/deformity/CSF (ears/nose)/mouth clear/cyanosis?
Eyes:	- Pupils: equal & react to light (PEARL)/inner eyelid color?
Chest:	- Wounds/penetrating object? - Pain (with/without rib spring)?
Abdomen:	- Wounds/penetrating object? - Pain/guarding/rigidity (with/without gentle pushing)?
Extremities:	- Wounds/deformity/tenderness (compare 2 sides)? - pulses? - capillary refill?
Spinal cord:	- Finger/toe wiggle? - Touch finger/toe for sensation? - Hand squeeze/foot push?

Medical Alert Tag?

The secondary survey is done to discover problems that do not pose an immediate threat to life but may do so if they remain uncorrected. The secondary survey can detect less easily noticed injuries that can be aggravated by mishandling and can find problems which the EMS personnel and other medical authorities might find useful. If a victim with a spinal injury is mishandled, he or she could suffer spinal damage, leading to paralysis. Also, a closed fracture can become an open fracture if not immobilized.

The secondary survey is a head-to-toe examination. Start by examining the victim's head, then neck, trunk, and extremities, looking for abnormalities such as swelling, discoloration, and tenderness, which might indicate an unseen injury. (See Table 2.1)

Putting It All Together

The victim assessment will be influenced by whether the victim is suffering from a medical problem or an injury, whether the victim is conscious or unconscious, and whether life-threatening conditions are present. Remember to first conduct a primary survey and correct any problems it uncovers before going on to the secondary survey.

Medical Alert Tag

A medical alert emblem tag worn as a necklace or as a bracelet attracts attention in an emergency situation. These tags contain the wearer's medical problem and a 24-hour telephone number to call in case of an emergency. Do *not* remove a medical alert tag from an injured or sick person.

Calling the Emergency Medical Services (EMS) System for Help*

In many communities, to receive emergency assistance of every kind you just dial 9–1–1. Check to see if this is true in your community. An emergency number should be listed on the inside cover of your telephone directory.

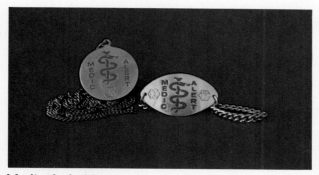

Medical alert tag

To receive the best emergency medical help fast, you should keep a list of phone numbers for the following services near your telephone.

1. *The rescue squad.* Often part of the local fire department, these specially trained paramedics are likely to respond swiftly and competently.

2. *The police.* They may or may not be able to respond with medically trained personnel; however, they can get someone to the hospital quickly.

3. *Ambulance service.* Some services have trained paramedics; others do not.

4. *Your doctor.* Your own doctor may not be available, but he or she should be alerted if an emergency has occurred.

5. *Poison control center.* In some communities, this service will give information to doctors only. Call before an emergency occurs to find out.

Give the following information over the phone:

1. *The victim's location.* Give city or town, street name, and street number. Give names of intersecting streets or roads and other landmarks if possible. Describe the building. The victim's location may be the single most important information you can provide.

2. *Your phone number.* This information is required not only to help prevent false calls but, more importantly, to allow the center to call back for additional information.

3. *What has happened.* Tell the nature of the emergency (traffic accident, heart attack, dog bite, and so on).

4. *Number of persons needing help and any special conditions.* Tell the number of people involved. Tell about any special problems, such as several flights of stairs and no elevators, or the presence of a guard dog.

5. *Condition of the victim(s).* Tell about such things as no breathing or pulse, severe bleeding, unconsciousness.

6. *What is being done for the victim(s).* Tell about CPR, how the bleeding is being controlled, and so on.

Always be the last to hang up the phone. The EMS system dispatcher may need to ask more questions about how to find you. They may also tell you what to do until help arrives.

Speak slowly and clearly. Shouting is difficult to understand.

According to the National Emergency Number Association, 75 percent of the population and 25 percent of the geographic area in the United States have 9-1-1 coverage. Record your local community emergency telephone numbers and other information on this book's back cover.

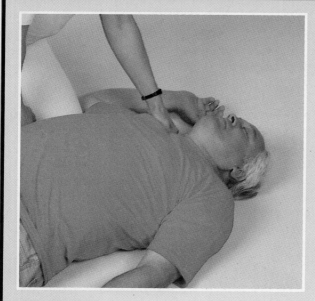

Responsive?

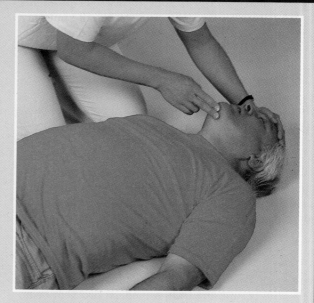

A = Airway open?

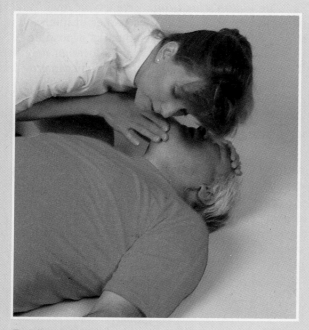

B = Breathing?

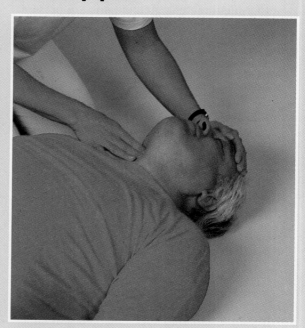

C = Circulation at carotid pulse?

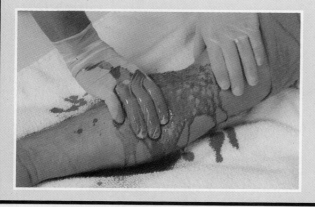

H = Hemorrhage—severe bleeding?

3

Basic Life Support*

What is CPR?

Cardiopulmonary resuscitation (CPR) combines rescue breathing (also known as mouth-to-mouth breathing) and external chest compressions. *Cardio* refers to the heart and *pulmonary* refers to the lungs. *Resuscitation* refers to revive. Proper and prompt CPR serves as a holding action by providing oxygen to the brain and heart until advanced cardiac life support (ACLS) can be provided.

Need for CPR Training

Heart disease causes more than half the deaths in North America. About two-thirds of these deaths are from heart attacks, and more than half of these were dead on arrival (DOA) at a hospital. Sudden death related to heart attacks is the most prominent medical emergency in the United States today.

It is possible that a large number of these deaths could be prevented by prompt action to provide rapid entry into the EMS system, prompt CPR, and early defibrillation. CPR can save heart attack victims, and it can also save lives in cases of drowning, suffocation, electrocution, and drug overdose. Use CPR any time a victim's breathing and heart have stopped. Use rescue breathing whenever there is a pulse but no breathing.

When to Start CPR

Trained people need to be able to:

- Recognize the signs of cardiac arrest
- Provide CPR, and
- Call for the emergency medical services (EMS).

Most people suffering a fatal heart attack die within two hours of the first signs and symptoms of the attack.

Activate the EMS system and start CPR as soon as possible! Victims have a good chance of surviving if:

- CPR is started within the first four minutes of heart stoppage, and
- They receive advanced cardiac life support within the next four minutes.

Brain damage begins after four to six minutes and is certain after ten minutes when no CPR is given.

Signs of Successful CPR

Successful CPR refers to correct CPR performance, not victim survival. Even with successful CPR, most victims will not survive unless they receive advanced cardiac life support (e.g., defibrillation, oxygen, and drug therapy). CPR serves as a holding action until such medical care can be provided. Early bystander CPR (started in less than four minutes after cardiac arrest) coupled with an EMS system with advanced cardiac life support capability (within eight minutes) can increase survival chances to more than 40 percent.

Check CPR's effectiveness by:

- Watching chest rise and fall with each rescue breath

*Based on the 1992 American Heart Association, Guidelines for Cardiopulmonary Resuscitation and Emergency Cardiac Care, JAMA, 1992; 268:2172

TABLE 3-1 Chances of Survival (Survival Rate %)				
		Time Until Advanced Cardiac Life Support Begins		
		<8 min.	8–16 min.	>16 min.
Time Until Basic Life Support (CPR)	<4 min.	43%	19%	10%
	4–8 min.	27%	19%	6%
	>8 min.	N/A	7%	0%

Source: National Ski Patrol, based upon Eisenberg, et. al., JAMA, 1979; 241:1905–1907.

7

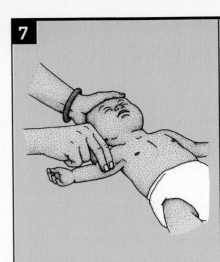

Check for pulse
- Maintain head-tilt with hand nearest head on forehead.
- Feel for pulse located on the inside of the upper arm between the elbow and armpit (known as the brachial).
- Press gently with 2 fingers on inside of arm closest to you.
- Place thumb of same hand on outside of infant's upper arm.

8

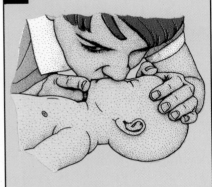

Perform rescue procedures based upon your pulse check

If there is a pulse
Give rescue breaths (mouth-to-mouth resuscitation) every 3 seconds. Use the same techniques for rescue breathing found in Step 6 but only give one breath. Every minute (20 breaths) stop and check the pulse to make sure there is a pulse. Continue until:

- Infant starts breathing on his or her own.

OR
- Trained help, such as emergency medical technicians (EMTs), arrive and relieve you.

OR
- You are completely exhausted.

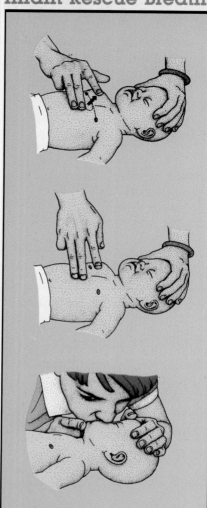

If there is no pulse, give CPR:

- Locate fingers' position

    1. Maintain head-tilt

    2. Imagine a line connecting the nipples

    3. Place 3 fingers on sternum with index finger touching but below imaginary nipple line.

    4. Raise your index finger and use other 2 fingers for compression. If you feel the notch at the end of the sternum, move your fingers up a little.

- Give 5 compressions

    1. Do 5 chest compressions at rate of 100 per minute or count as you push down, "one, two, three, four, five."

    2. Press sternum ½ to 1 inch or about ⅓ to ½ of the depth of the chest.

    3. Keep fingers pointing across the infant's chest away from you. Keep fingers in contact with infant's chest.

    4. Maintain head-tilt with hand nearest head on forehead.

- Give 1 breath

- Complete 20 cycles of 5 compressions and one breath (takes about 1 minute) and check the pulse. If rescuer is alone, activate the EMS system. If there is no pulse, restart CPR with chest compressions. Recheck the pulse every few minutes. If there is a pulse, give rescue breathing.

- Give CPR until:

    Infant revives.

    OR

    Trained help, such as emergency medical technicians (EMTs), arrives and relieves you.

    OR

    You are completely exhausted.

Conscious Infant Foreign Body Airway Obstruction (Choking)

	If infant is conscious and cannot cough, cry, or breathe . . .
1	**Give up to 5 back blows** ■ Hold infant's head and neck with 1 hand by firmly holding infant's jaw between your thumb and fingers. ■ Lay infant face down over your forearm with head lower than his/her chest. Brace your forearm and infant against your thigh. ■ Give up to 5 distinct and separate back blows between shoulder blades with the heel of your hand.
2	**Give up to 5 chest thrusts** ■ Support the back of infant's head. ■ Sandwich infant between your hands and arms, turn on back, with head lower than his/her chest. Small rescuers may need to support infant on their lap. ■ Imagine a line connecting infant's nipples. ■ Place 3 fingers on sternum with your ring finger next to imaginary nipple line on the infant's feet side. ■ Lift your ring finger off chest. If you feel the notch at the end of the sternum, move your fingers up a little. ■ Give up to 5 separate and distinct thrusts with index and middle fingers on sternum in a manner similar to CPR chest compressions, but at a slower rate. ■ Keep fingers in contact with chest between chest thrusts.

3	**Repeat**
	1. Up to 5 back blows
	2. Up to 5 chest thrusts until:
	    ■ infant becomes unconscious, or
	    ■ object is expelled and infant begins to breathe or coughs forcefully

Unconscious Infant with Foreign Body Airway Obstruction (Choking)

	If infant is motionless . . .
1	**Check responsiveness** ■ If head or neck injury is suspected, move only if absolutely necessary. ■ Tap or gently shake infant's shoulder.
2	**Send bystander, if available, to activate the EMS system. If alone, resuscitate for one minute before activating the EMS system.**
3	**Give 2 slow breaths** ■ Open the airway with head-tilt/chin-lift. ■ Seal your mouth over infant's mouth and nose. ■ Give 2 slow breaths (1 to 1½ seconds each) If first 2 breaths do not go in, retilt the head and try 2 more slow breaths.
4	**Give up to 5 back blows** ■ Hold infant's head and neck with 1 hand by firmly holding infant's jaw between your thumb and fingers. ■ Lay infant face down over your forearm with head lower than his/her chest. Brace your forearm and infant against your thigh. ■ Give up to 5 distinct and separate back blows between shoulder blades with the heel of your hand.

5

Give up to 5 chest thrusts
- Support the back of infant's head.
- Sandwich infant between your hands and arms, turn on back, with head lower than his/her chest. Small rescuers may need to support infant on their lap.
- Imagine a line connecting infant's nipples.
- Place 3 fingers on sternum with your ring finger next to imaginary nipple line on the infant's feet side.
- Lift your ring finger off chest. If you feel the notch at the end of the sternum, move your fingers up a little.
- Give up to 5 separate and distinct thrusts with index and middle fingers on sternum in a manner similar to CPR chest compressions, but at a slower rate.
- Keep fingers in contact with chest between chest thrusts.

6

Check mouth for foreign object
- Grasp both tongue and jaw between your thumb and fingers and lift up.
- If object is seen, remove with a finger sweep by sliding your little finger of the other hand alongside cheek to base of tongue using a hooking action.
- Do not try to remove an unseen object (known as a "blind finger sweep").
- Do not push object deeper.

7

Repeat
1. 2 slow breaths (retilt head and try 2 more breaths if first 2 are unsuccessful)
2. Up to 5 back blows
3. Up to 5 chest thrusts
4. Check mouth for foreign object (if object is seen, use finger sweep)

Repeat steps until object is expelled or EMS system arrives.
If you are alone and after 1 minute the object has not been expelled then take infant with you and call the EMS system.

4

Shock

Most injuries involve some degree of shock. Shock occurs when the circulatory system fails to deliver oxygenated blood to every part of the body.

Types of Shock

Several types of shock exist; first aiders usually concern themselves mainly with these three types: hypovolemic, fainting, and anaphylactic shock (the latter is better known as a severe allergic reaction).

Hypovolemic

Hypovolemic shock results from blood or fluid loss. If related to blood loss it is best known as hemorrhagic shock.

Signs and Symptoms

- Pale or bluish skin, nailbed, and lips
- Slow capillary filling time
- Cool, wet (clammy) skin; heavy sweating
- Rapid breathing and pulse
- Dilated (enlarged) pupils
- Dull, sunken look to the eyes
- Thirst
- Nausea and vomiting
- Loss of consciousness in severe shock

Even if signs and symptoms have not appeared in a severely injured victim, treat for shock. **First aiders can prevent shock; they cannot reverse it.**

Fainting

Fainting involves a sudden, temporary loss of consciousness. It occurs when the brain's blood flow is interrupted. Numerous causes account for the interrupted blood flow.

Signs and Symptoms

Fainting may occur suddenly or may be preceded by warning signs including any or all of the following:

- Dizziness
- "Seeing spots"
- Nausea
- Paleness
- Sweating

Severe Allergic Reaction (Anaphylactic Shock)

Allergies are usually thought of as causing rashes, itching, or some other short-term discomfort that disappears when the offending agent is removed from contact with the allergic person. There is, however, a more powerful reaction to substances ordinarily eaten or injected called anaphylactic shock, which can occur within minutes and even in some cases within seconds. Such a reaction can cause death if not treated immediately.

The severe allergic response (anaphylactic shock) is triggered by contact with a substance that the individual has previously encountered and the body has identified as an enemy, causing the development of antibodies called IgE. The antibodies, or body defenders, later come in contact with the offending substance and release chemicals (e.g., histamine) that attack the lungs, blood vessels, intestine, and skin. **It is a life-threatening situation!** About 60–80 percent of anaphylactic deaths are caused by an inability to breathe because swollen airway passages obstruct airflow to the lungs. The second most common cause of anaphylactic deaths—about 24 percent—is shock, brought on by insufficient blood circulating through the body.

Signs and Symptoms

One or all of these signs and symptoms may appear:

- Coughing, sneezing, or wheezing
- Difficult breathing
- Tightness and swelling in the throat
- Tightness in the chest
- Severe itching, burning, rash, or hives
- Swollen face, tongue, mouth
- Nausea and vomiting
- Dizziness
- Abdominal cramps
- Blueness (cyanosis) around the lips and mouth
- Unconsciousness

■ HYPOVOLEMIC SHOCK ■

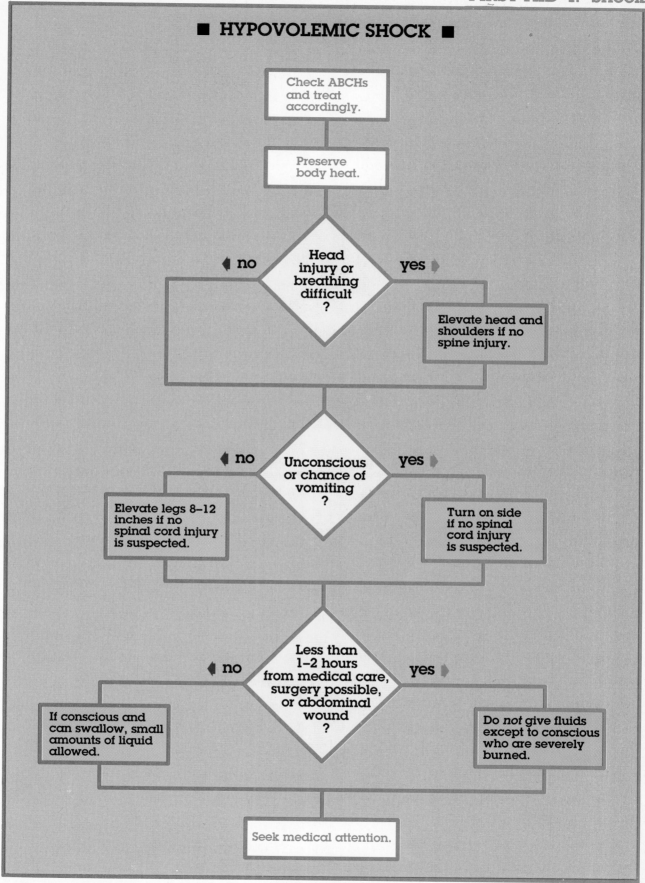

Check ABCHs and treat accordingly.

↓

Preserve body heat.

↓

Head injury or breathing difficult?

◀ no   yes ▶

Elevate head and shoulders if no spine injury.

Unconscious or chance of vomiting?

◀ no   yes ▶

Elevate legs 8–12 inches if no spinal cord injury is suspected.

Turn on side if no spinal cord injury is suspected.

Less than 1–2 hours from medical care, surgery possible, or abdominal wound?

◀ no   yes ▶

If conscious and can swallow, small amounts of liquid allowed.

Do *not* give fluids except to conscious who are severely burned.

Seek medical attention.

■ FAINTING ■

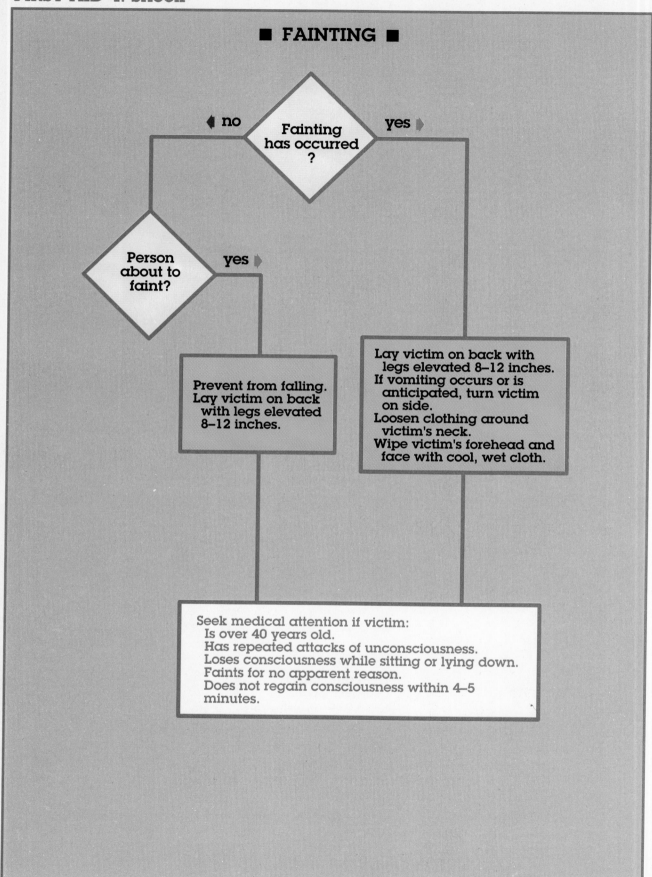

◀ no   **Fainting has occurred ?**   yes ▶

Person about to faint?   yes ▶

Prevent from falling. Lay victim on back with legs elevated 8–12 inches.

Lay victim on back with legs elevated 8–12 inches.
If vomiting occurs or is anticipated, turn victim on side.
Loosen clothing around victim's neck.
Wipe victim's forehead and face with cool, wet cloth.

Seek medical attention if victim:
Is over 40 years old.
Has repeated attacks of unconsciousness.
Loses consciousness while sitting or lying down.
Faints for no apparent reason.
Does not regain consciousness within 4–5 minutes.

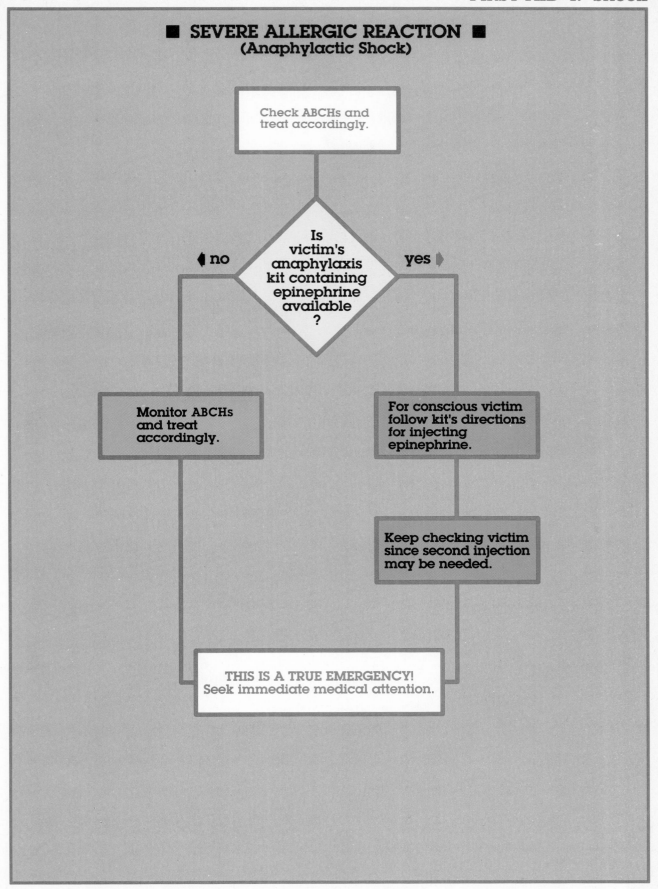

■ SEVERE ALLERGIC REACTION ■
(Anaphylactic Shock)

Check ABCHs and treat accordingly.

Is victim's anaphylaxis kit containing epinephrine available?

no

yes

Monitor ABCHs and treat accordingly.

For conscious victim follow kit's directions for injecting epinephrine.

Keep checking victim since second injection may be needed.

THIS IS A TRUE EMERGENCY!
Seek immediate medical attention.

SKILL SCAN: Positioning the Shock Victim

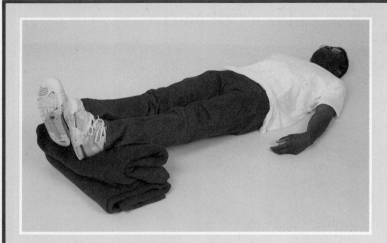

Usual shock position. Elevate the legs 8-12 inches. Do not lift the foot of bed or stretcher.

EXCEPTIONS:

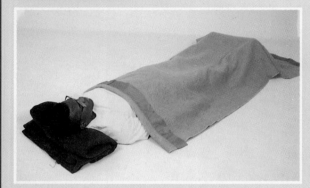

Elevate the head for injuries or stroke.

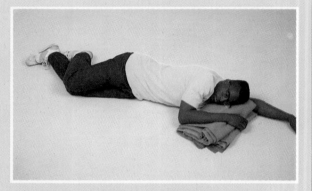

Lay an unconcious, semiconcious, or vomiting victim on his or her side.

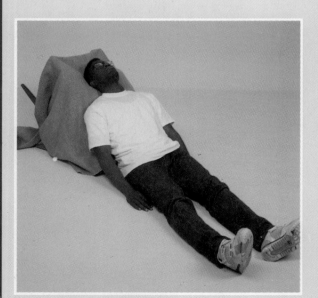

Use a semisitting position for those with breathing difficulties, chest injuries, or a heart attack.

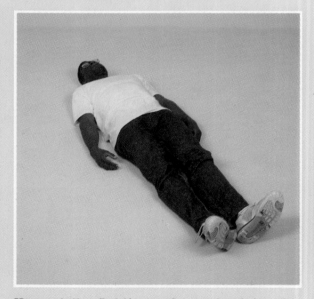

Keep victim flat if a neck or spine injury is suspected or victim has leg fractures.

Bleeding and Wounds

The average-sized adult has about six quarts of blood and can safely lose a pint during a blood donation. However, rapid blood loss of one quart or more can lead to shock and death. A child losing one pint is in extreme danger.

Blood can be lost from arteries, veins, or capillaries. Most bleeding involves more than one type of blood vessel. Blood from arteries is bright red and spurts. Arterial bleeding loses blood the fastest, is the most difficult to control, and is therefore the most dangerous.

Blood from a vein flows steadily and appears to be a darker red. Blood oozes slowly from capillaries. Though each blood vessel contains blood differing in shades of red, an inexperienced person may have difficulty detecting the difference. The two basic types of bleeding are external and internal.

External Bleeding

This type involves seeing blood coming from a wound. In most cases, bleeding stops after 5 to 10 minutes with proper first aid.

Internal Bleeding

Bleeding occurs when the skin is unbroken, and is not usually visible.

Signs and Symptoms

- Blood from the mouth (vomit, sputum) or rectum, or blood in the urine
- Nonmenstrual bleeding from the vagina
- Bruise or contusion
- Rapid pulse
- Cold and moist skin
- Dilated pupils
- Nausea and vomiting
- Pain, tender, rigid, bruised abdomen
- Fractured ribs or bruises on chest

Animal and Human Bites

Animal bites rarely cause lethal bleeding, but they can produce significant damage. Sixty to 90% of the animal bites in the United States come from dogs. The annual

TABLE 5-1 Types of Open Wounds

Type	Cause(s)	Signs and Symptoms	First Aid
Abrasion (scrape)	Rubbing or scraping	Only skin surface affected Little bleeding	Remove all debris. Wash away from wound with soap and water.
Incision (cut)	Sharp objects	Smooth edges of wound Severe bleeding	Control bleeding. Wash wound.
Laceration (tearing)	Blunt object tearing skin	Veins and arteries can be affected Severe bleeding Danger of infection	Control bleeding. Wash wound.
Puncture (stab)	Sharp pointed object pierces skin	Wound is narrow and deep into veins and arteries Embedded objects Danger of infection	Do not remove impaled objects.
Avulsion (torn off)	Machinery, Explosives	Tissue torn off or left hanging Severe bleeding	Control bleeding. Take avulsed part to medical facility.

Bloodborne pathogens are disease-causing microorganisms that may be present in human blood. They may be transmitted with any exposure to blood. Two significant pathogens are Hepatitis B Virus (HBV) and Human Immunodeficiency Virus (HIV). A number of bloodborne diseases other than HIV and HBV exist, such as Hepatitis C, Hepatitis D, and syphilis. Other body fluids may also spread bloodborne pathogens.

The HBV attacks the liver. HBV is very infectious and can cause:

■ Active hepatitis B—a flu-like illness that can last for months

■ A chronic carrier state—the person may have no symptoms, but can pass HBV to others

■ Cirrhosis, liver cancer, and death

Fortunately, vaccines are available to prevent HBV infection. Even if you are vaccinated against HBV, you must treat all blood and certain human body fluids as if they are known to be infected with bloodborne pathogens (known as the "universal precautions").

HIV causes AIDS (Acquired Immune Deficiency Syndrome). HIV attacks the immune system, making the body less able to fight off infections. In most cases, these infections eventually prove fatal. At present there is no vaccine to prevent infection and no known cure for AIDS.

Use personal protective equipment whenever possible while giving first aid:

1. Keep open wounds covered with dressings to prevent contact with blood.

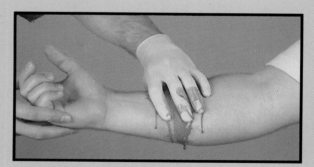

Whenever possible, use gloves as a barrier.

2. All first aid kits should have several pairs of latex gloves. Use these gloves in every situation involving blood or other body fluids.

3. If latex gloves are not available, use the most waterproof material available or extra gauze dressings to form a barrier.

4. Whenever possible, use a mouth-to-barrier device for protection when doing rescue breathing. Every first aid kit should have one. While saliva is not considered a high risk, there may be blood in the mouth.

A person exposed to blood or other body fluids should:

1. Wash the exposed area immediately with soap and running water. Scrub vigorously with lots of lather.

2. Report the incident promptly, according to your workplace policy.

3. Get medical help, treatment and counseling. If your workplace is covered by OSHA's Bloodborne Standards, ask about getting a confidential medical evaluation, testing, counseling, and treatment.

4. Ask about HBV globulin (HBIG) if you haven't had the HBV vaccine. It can provide short-term protection. It's followed by vaccination againts HBV.

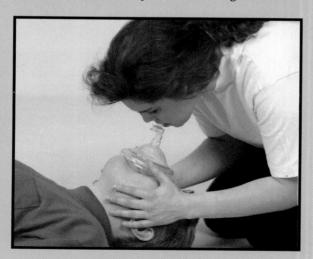

Pocket face mask, one-way valve.

number of dog bites has been estimated to be between one and two million.

Animal bites of all kinds account for about one percent of all hospital emergency department visits. About one bite in 10 needs stitches, but all bites require complete cleaning, which may be impossible for a first aider.

A dog's mouth may carry more than 60 different species of bacteria, some of which are very dangerous to humans (e.g., rabies). Human, cat, and other animal bites are equally contaminated and dangerous.

Human bites can cause very serious injury. The human mouth contains a wide range of bacteria, and the likelihood of infection is greater from a human bite than from other warm-blooded animals.

■ BLEEDING ■

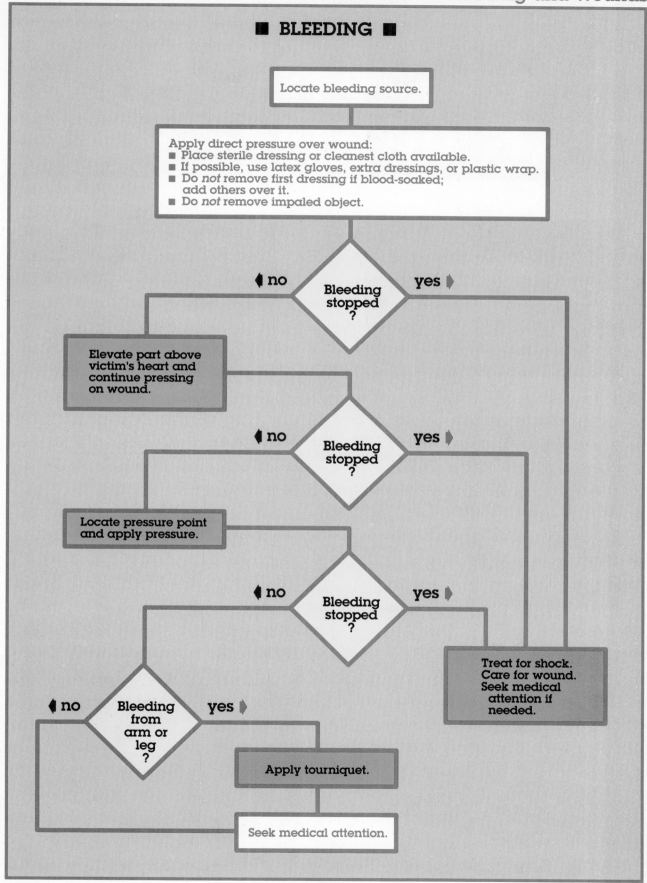

Locate bleeding source.

Apply direct pressure over wound:
- Place sterile dressing or cleanest cloth available.
- If possible, use latex gloves, extra dressings, or plastic wrap.
- Do *not* remove first dressing if blood-soaked; add others over it.
- Do *not* remove impaled object.

Bleeding stopped?

no → Elevate part above victim's heart and continue pressing on wound.

yes →

Bleeding stopped?

no → Locate pressure point and apply pressure.

yes →

Bleeding stopped?

no → **Bleeding from arm or leg?**

yes →

Treat for shock. Care for wound. Seek medical attention if needed.

Bleeding from arm or leg?

no →

yes → Apply tourniquet.

Seek medical attention.

■ ABDOMINAL INJURIES ■

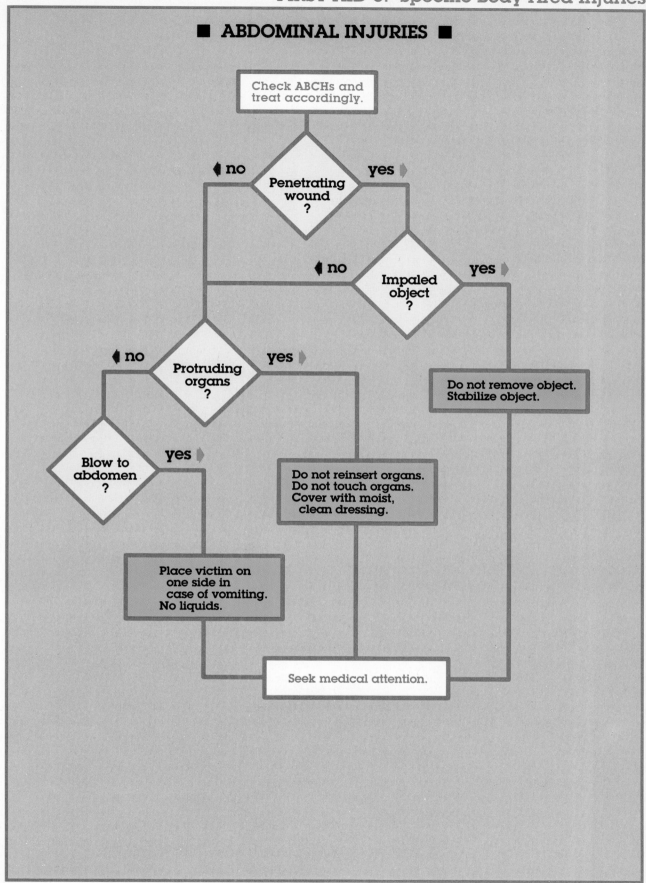

■ BLISTERS ■

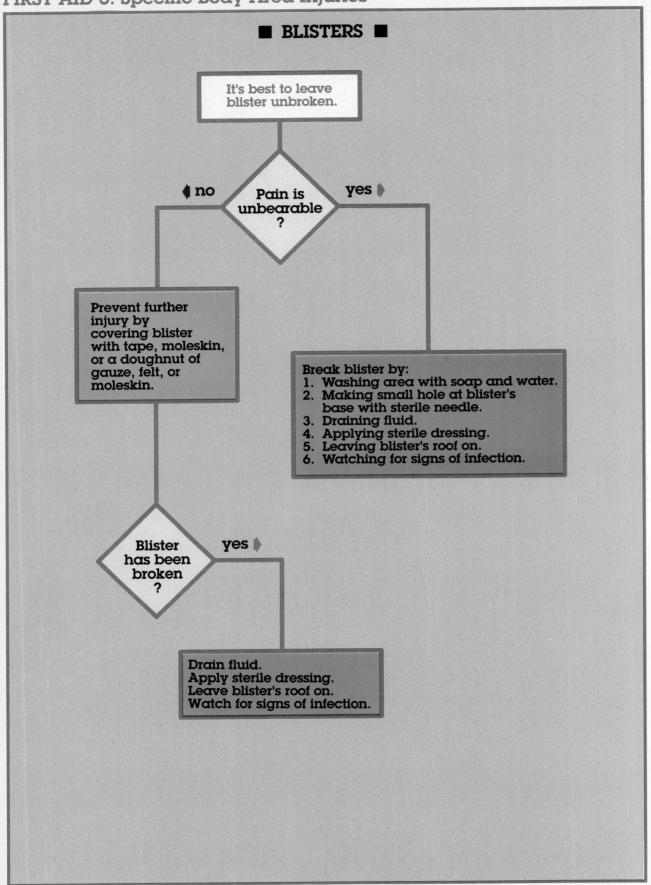

It's best to leave blister unbroken.

Pain is unbearable?

no ◀ | yes ▶

no: Prevent further injury by covering blister with tape, moleskin, or a doughnut of gauze, felt, or moleskin.

yes: Break blister by:
1. Washing area with soap and water.
2. Making small hole at blister's base with sterile needle.
3. Draining fluid.
4. Applying sterile dressing.
5. Leaving blister's roof on.
6. Watching for signs of infection.

Blister has been broken?

yes ▶

Drain fluid.
Apply sterile dressing.
Leave blister's roof on.
Watch for signs of infection.

7
Poisoning

Swallowed Poison

A poison is a relatively small amount of any substance (solid, liquid, or gas) that when swallowed, inhaled, absorbed, or injected can by its chemical action damage tissue or adversely change organ function and thus can affect health or cause death.

Deaths by swallowing poisoning have dramatically decreased in recent years, particularly in children under the age of five. Despite this reduction, nonfatal poisoning remains a major cause of hospital admissions and emergency room care. For every poisoning death among children under the age of five, 80,000 to 90,000 nonfatal cases are seen in emergency rooms and about 20,000 children are hospitalized.

Signs and Symptoms

- Abdominal pain and cramping
- Nausea or vomiting
- Diarrhea
- Burns, odor, stains around and in mouth
- Drowsiness or unconsciousness
- Poison containers or plants nearby

Determine the critical information, which includes:

1. *Who?* Age and size of the victim
2. *What?* Type of poison swallowed
3. *How much?* A taste, half a bottle, etc.
4. *How?* Circumstances
5. *When?* Time taken

Contact the poison control center, hospital emergency department, or a physician immediately. Some poisons produce little damage until hours later, while others do damage immediately. More than 70% of poisonings can be treated through instructions taken over the telephone. Otherwise, victims should be transported to a medical facility.

Insect Stings

For a severely allergic person, a single sting may be fatal within 15 minutes. Although accounts exist of individuals who have survived some 2,000 stings, generally 500 or more stings will kill people who are not allergic to stinging insects.

Some experts report that 1% of all children and 4% of adults have such an allergy. An estimated 50–100 sting-related deaths occur yearly. The number of cases may actually be higher but not reported as involving insect stings because they are mistaken for hearts attacks or naturally caused death.

Signs and Symptoms

- *Usual reactions.* Momentary pain, redness around sting site, itching, heat
- *Worrisome reactions.* Skin flush, hives, localized swelling of lips or tongue, "tickle" in throat, wheezing, abdominal cramps, diarrhea
- *Life-threatening reactions.* Bluish or grayish skin color (cyanosis), seizures, unconsciousness, inability to breathe due to swelling of vocal cords

Those who have had a reaction to an insect sting should be instructed in self-treatment so they can protect themselves from severe reactions. They should also be advised to purchase a medical alert bracelet or necklace identifying them as insect-allergic.

Snakebites

Throughout the world about 50,000 people die each year from snakebite. In the United States, of the 40,000 to 50,000 annually bitten, over 7,000 are bitten by poisonous snakes. Amazingly, only a dozen Americans die each year.

Of the many different snake species, only four in the United States are poisonous: rattlesnake, copperhead, water moccasin, and coral snake. The first three are known as pit vipers. They have three common characteristics:

- Triangular, flat head wider than its neck
- Elliptical pupils (e.g., cat's eye)
- Heat-sensitive "pit" located between each eye and nostril

The coral snake is small and very colorful, with a series of bright red, yellow, and black bands around its body. Every other band is yellow. A black snout also marks the coral snake.

Pit Vipers

(rattlesnake, copperhead, water moccasin)

Signs and Symptoms

- Severe burning pain at the bite site
- Two small puncture wounds about 1/2 inch apart (some cases may have only one puncture wound)
- Swelling (happens within 5 minutes and can involve an entire extremity)
- Discoloration and blood-filled blisters
- In severe cases: nausea, vomiting, sweating, weakness
- No venom injected into the victim in about 25% of all poisonous snakebite cases, only fang and tooth wounds

Most snakebites occur within a few hours of a medical facility where antivenin is available. Bites showing no sign of venom injection require only a possible tetanus shot and care of the bite wounds (in the absence of pain or swelling).

Controversy exists about proper first aid procedures for snakebite.

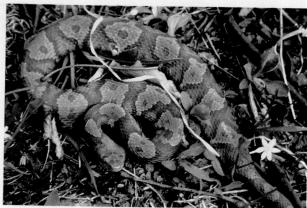

Copperhead snake

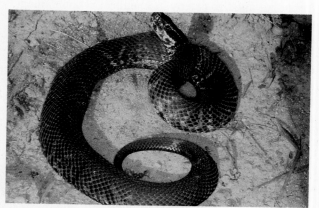

Cottonmouth water moccasin

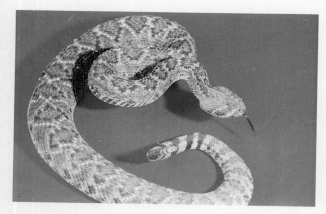

Rattlesnake

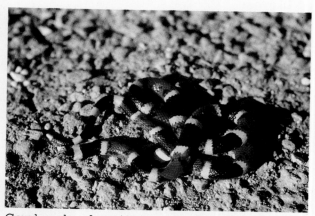

Coral snake, America's most poisonous snake

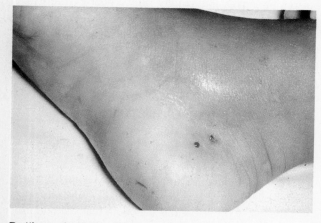

Rattlesnake bite. Note two fang marks.

Spider Bites

Two spiders, the black widow and the brown recluse, can be deadly.

Black Widow Spider

The black widow spider is found throughout the world. A red spot (often in the shape of an hourglass) on the abdomen identifies the female—she is the one that

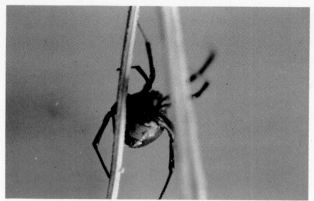

Black widow spider. Note red hour-glass configuration on abdomen.

bites. Females have a glossy black body. By volume, black widow spider venom is more deadly than the rattlesnake's, but it is injected in much smaller amounts.

Signs and Symptoms

Determining whether a person has been bitten by a black widow spider is difficult.

- A sharp pinprick of the spider's bite may be felt, although some victims are not even aware of the bite. In no more than 15 minutes, a dull, numbing pain develops in the bitten extremity.
- Faint red bite marks appear.
- Muscle stiffness and cramps occur next, usually affecting the abdomen when the bite is in the lower part of the body or legs, and affecting the shoulders, back, or chest when the bite is on the upper body or arms.
- Headache, chills, fever, heavy sweating, dizziness, nausea, vomiting, and severe abdominal pain afflict the victim.

Brown Recluse Spider

The brown recluse spider has a brown, possibly purplish, violin-shaped figure on its back. Brown recluse bites are rarely fatal, except for hypersensitive people or for children, the elderly, and those with chronic health problems.

Signs and Symptoms

- The initial pain felt may be slight enough to be overlooked.
- A blister at the bite site, along with redness and swelling, appears after several hours.
- Pain, which may remain mild but can become severe, develops within two to eight hours at the bite site.
- Fever, weakness, vomiting, joint pain, and a rash may occur.

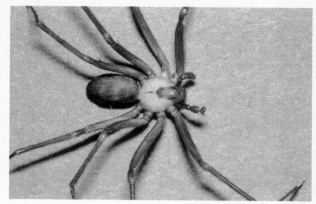

Brown recluse spider. Note violin or fiddle configuration on back.

- An ulcer forms within a week. Gangrene may develop in some cases.

Tarantula Spider

More menacing-looking than black widow and brown recluse spiders, the tarantula has a bite that rarely produces symptoms other than mild to moderate pain.

Scorpion Stings

Death from scorpion stings in the United States is rare; children are at greatest risk. A scorpion's sting causes immediate pain and burning around the sting site, followed by numbness or tingling. Severe cases may include paralysis, spasms, or respiratory difficulties.

Tick Bites

Most tick bites are harmless, though ticks can carry serious diseases (e.g., Lyme disease, Rocky Mountain spotted fever, Colorado tick fever). Ticks should be removed as soon as possible.

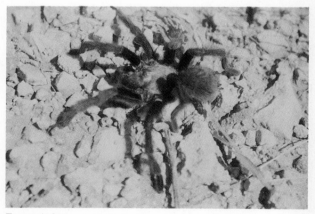

Tarantula

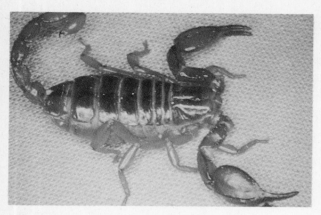
Scorpion

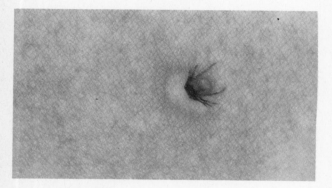
Tick embedded

Poison Ivy, Oak, and Sumac

Poison ivy, oak, and sumac plants cause contact dermatitis or an allergic reaction in about 90% of all adults. Most people cannot recognize these plants. To test a plant for poison, use the "black spot test." Perform this test by crushing the suspected plant's leaf. The sap of poison ivy or oak turns dark brown in 10 minutes and black in one day. Actually, more than 60 plants can cause an allergic reaction, but the three named above are by far the most common offenders.

Allergic people may come in contact with the juice of these plants from their clothes or shoes, from pet fur, or from smoke of burning plants. No one can develop the dermatitis by touching the fluid from blisters, since that fluid does not contain the oleoresin that comes from the juice of these poisonous plants.

Signs and Symptoms

- **Mild.** Some itching
- **Mild to moderate.** Itching and redness
- **Moderate.** Itching, redness, and swelling
- **Severe.** Itching, redness, swelling, and blisters

Severity is important but so is the amount of skin affected. The greater the skin involvement, the greater the need for medical attention. A day or two is the usual time between contact and the onset of the above signs and symptoms.

Carbon Monoxide

Victims of carbon monoxide (CO) are often unaware of its presence. The gas is invisible, tasteless, odorless, and nonirritating.

Carbon monoxide produces its toxicity due to several factors. CO becomes tightly bound to hemoglobin (red blood cells) that carries oxygen. With conscious victims it takes four to five hours with ordinary air (21% oxygen) or 30–40 minutes with 100% oxygen to reverse CO's effects. When CO levels in the air are high, the level of oxygen is probably low.

Signs and Symptoms

It is difficult to tell if a person is a victim of carbon monoxide poisoning. Sometimes, a complaint of having the flu is really a symptom of carbon monoxide poisoning.

- Headache
- Ringing in the ears (tinnitus)
- Angina (chest pain)
- Muscle weakness
- Nausea and vomiting
- Dizziness and visual changes (blurred or double vision)
- Unconsciousness
- Breathing and cardiac failure

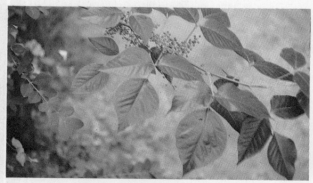
Poison ivy, found in all 48 contiguous U.S. states

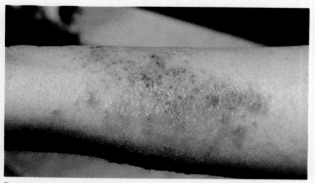
Poison ivy dermatitis

■ SWALLOWED POISON ■

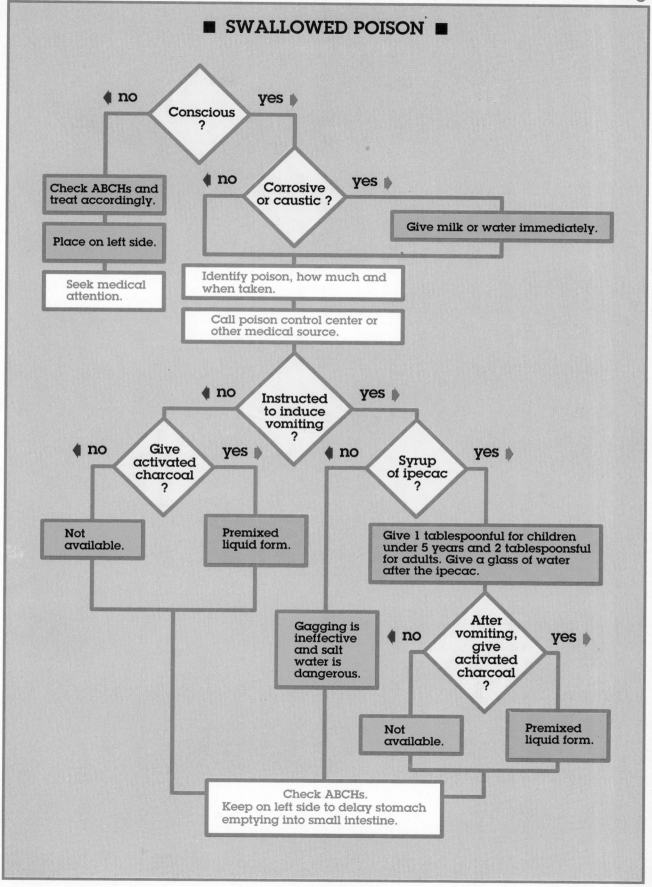

no ◄ **Conscious ?** ► yes

Check ABCHs and treat accordingly.

Place on left side.

Seek medical attention.

no ◄ **Corrosive or caustic ?** ► yes

Give milk or water immediately.

Identify poison, how much and when taken.

Call poison control center or other medical source.

no ◄ **Instructed to induce vomiting ?** ► yes

no ◄ **Give activated charcoal ?** ► yes

Not available.

Premixed liquid form.

no ◄ **Syrup of ipecac ?** ► yes

Gagging is ineffective and salt water is dangerous.

Give 1 tablespoonful for children under 5 years and 2 tablespoonsful for adults. Give a glass of water after the ipecac.

no ◄ **After vomiting, give activated charcoal ?** ► yes

Not available.

Premixed liquid form.

Check ABCHs.
Keep on left side to delay stomach emptying into small intestine.

■ INSECT STINGS ■
(Flying Insects)

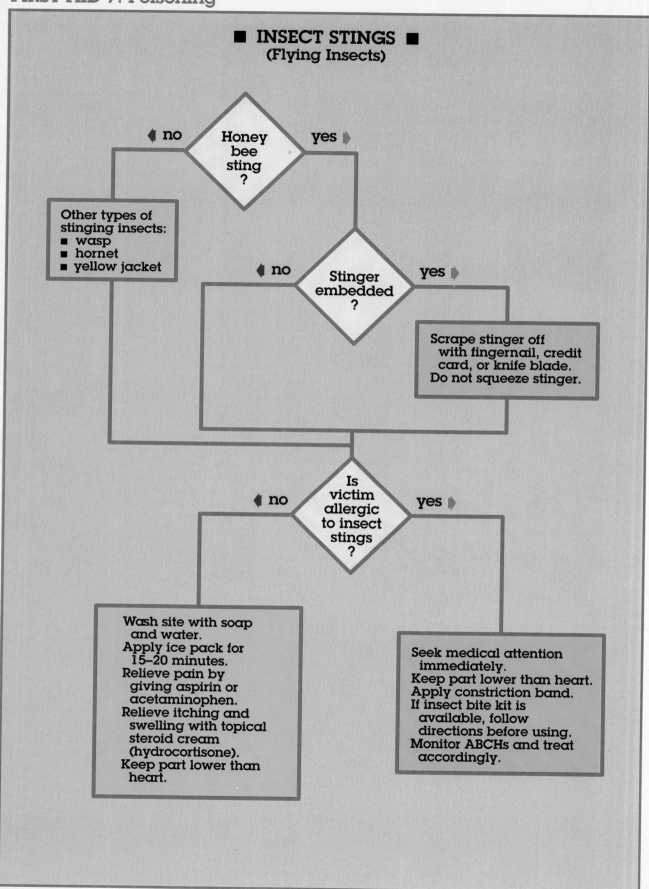

Honey bee sting ?

← no

yes ▶

Other types of stinging insects:
■ wasp
■ hornet
■ yellow jacket

Stinger embedded ?

← no

yes ▶

Scrape stinger off with fingernail, credit card, or knife blade. Do not squeeze stinger.

Is victim allergic to insect stings ?

← no

yes ▶

Wash site with soap and water.
Apply ice pack for 15–20 minutes.
Relieve pain by giving aspirin or acetaminophen.
Relieve itching and swelling with topical steroid cream (hydrocortisone).
Keep part lower than heart.

Seek medical attention immediately.
Keep part lower than heart.
Apply constriction band.
If insect bite kit is available, follow directions before using.
Monitor ABCHs and treat accordingly.

■ SNAKEBITES ■

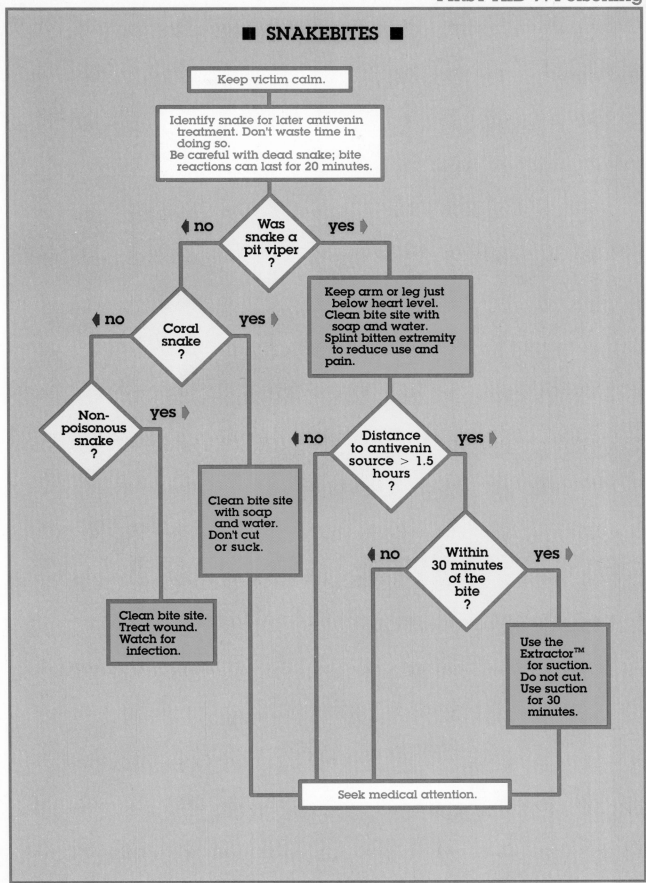

Keep victim calm.

Identify snake for later antivenin treatment. Don't waste time in doing so.
Be careful with dead snake; bite reactions can last for 20 minutes.

Was snake a pit viper ?

no ◄   yes ►

Keep arm or leg just below heart level.
Clean bite site with soap and water.
Splint bitten extremity to reduce use and pain.

Coral snake ?

no ◄   yes ►

Non-poisonous snake ?

yes ►

Clean bite site with soap and water. Don't cut or suck.

Distance to antivenin source > 1.5 hours ?

no ◄   yes ►

Within 30 minutes of the bite ?

no ◄   yes ►

Clean bite site. Treat wound. Watch for infection.

Use the Extractor™ for suction. Do not cut. Use suction for 30 minutes.

Seek medical attention.

■ SPIDER BITES AND SCORPION STINGS ■

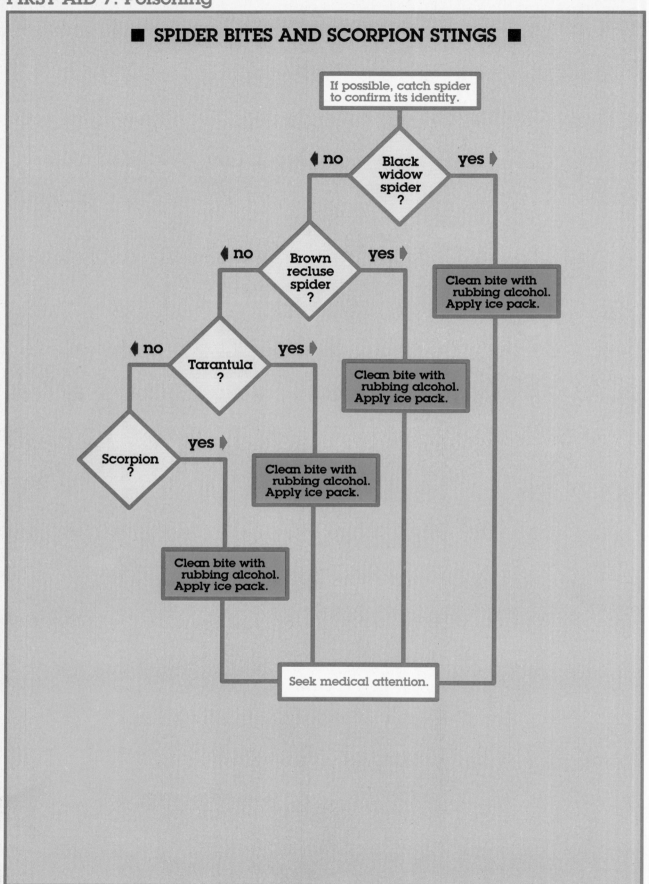

If possible, catch spider to confirm its identity.

Black widow spider ?
- no
- yes → Clean bite with rubbing alcohol. Apply ice pack.

Brown recluse spider ?
- no
- yes → Clean bite with rubbing alcohol. Apply ice pack.

Tarantula ?
- no
- yes → Clean bite with rubbing alcohol. Apply ice pack.

Scorpion ?
- yes → Clean bite with rubbing alcohol. Apply ice pack.

Seek medical attention.

■ TICK REMOVAL ■

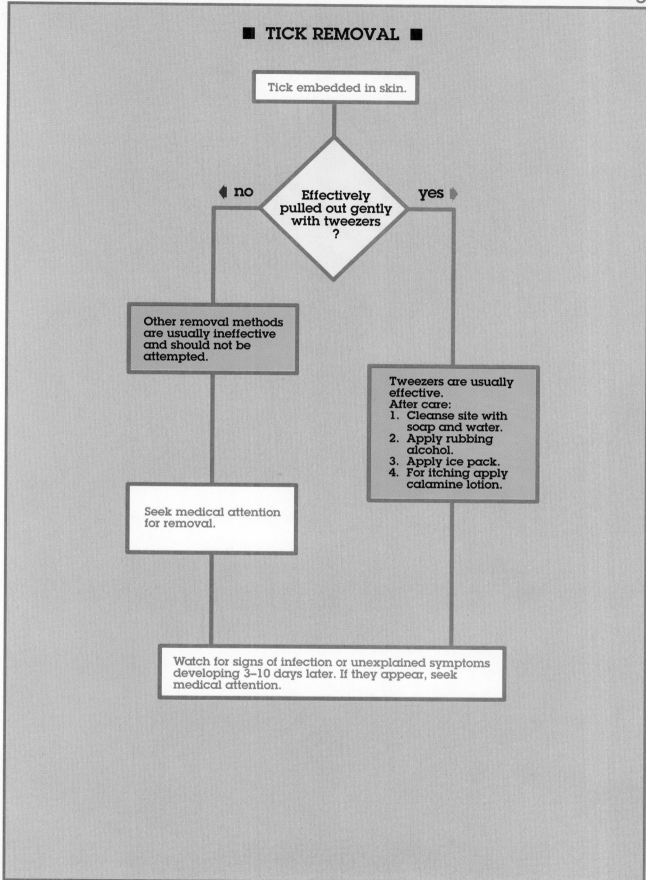

Tick embedded in skin.

◀ no | **Effectively pulled out gently with tweezers ?** | **yes ▶**

Other removal methods are usually ineffective and should not be attempted.

Tweezers are usually effective.
After care:
1. Cleanse site with soap and water.
2. Apply rubbing alcohol.
3. Apply ice pack.
4. For itching apply calamine lotion.

Seek medical attention for removal.

Watch for signs of infection or unexplained symptoms developing 3–10 days later. If they appear, seek medical attention.

■ POISON IVY ■

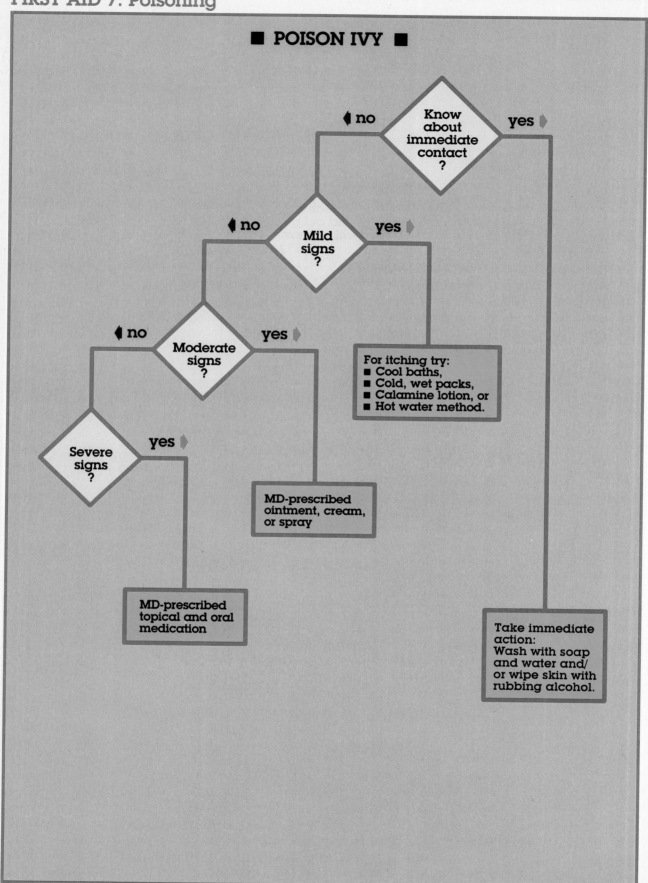

Know about immediate contact?

no / yes

Mild signs?

no / yes

Moderate signs?

no / yes

Severe signs?

yes

For itching try:
■ Cool baths,
■ Cold, wet packs,
■ Calamine lotion, or
■ Hot water method.

MD-prescribed ointment, cream, or spray

MD-prescribed topical and oral medication

Take immediate action:
Wash with soap and water and/or wipe skin with rubbing alcohol.

■ INHALED POISON ■

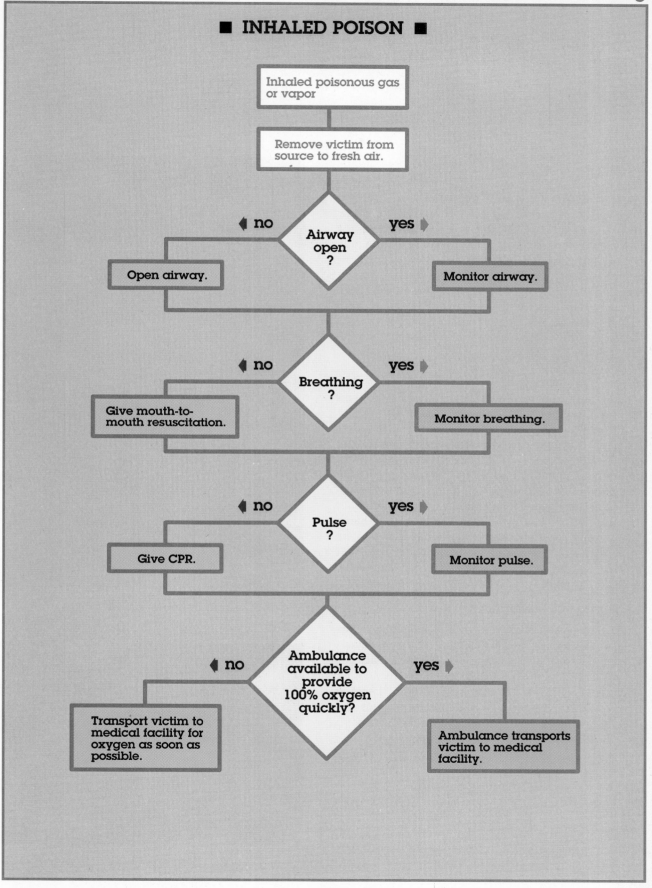

Inhaled poisonous gas or vapor

Remove victim from source to fresh air.

Airway open ?
- no → Open airway.
- yes → Monitor airway.

Breathing ?
- no → Give mouth-to-mouth resuscitation.
- yes → Monitor breathing.

Pulse ?
- no → Give CPR.
- yes → Monitor pulse.

Ambulance available to provide 100% oxygen quickly?
- no → Transport victim to medical facility for oxygen as soon as possible.
- yes → Ambulance transports victim to medical facility.

- **Exertional.** This type affects a healthy individual when strenuously working or playing in a warm environment.

Signs and Symptoms

- Loss of consciousness
- Hot skin. Victims do not sweat because the sweating mechanism is overwhelmed. Half the victims with exertional heat stroke may have sweat on the skin since they are progressing from heat exhaustion (having sweaty skin) into heat stroke.
- High body temperature
- Rapid pulse and breathing
- Weakness, dizziness, headache

Heat Exhaustion

Heat exhaustion results from either excessive perspiration or the inadequate replacement of water lost by sweating. It is less critical than heat stroke, but it requires prompt attention because it can progress to heat stroke if left untreated.

Signs and Symptoms

- Heavy sweating
- Weakness
- Fast pulse
- Normal body temperature
- Headache and dizziness
- Nausea and vomiting

Heat Cramps

Heat cramps are painful muscle spasms in the arms or legs. They may occur when an excessive amount of body fluid is lost through sweating. Controversy exists regarding what type of liquid to drink—plain water, a commercial sports drink, or a saltwater solution. The body loses more water than electrolytes (sodium, potassium, etc.) during exercise. Experts generally agree that the primary need for those sweating in hot environments is to replace the water lost from heavy sweating, rather than the electrolytes. However, mildly salted water (¼ to 1 level teaspoon in 1 quart of water) or electrolyte drink can be given.

Routine use of salt tablets to prevent heat cramps is no longer recommended since they can induce high blood pressure and hinder adjustment to heat.

Signs and Symptoms

- Severe cramping, usually affecting arms or legs
- Abdominal cramping

Heat Syncope

This condition resembles fainting and is usually self-correcting. Victims who are not nauseous can drink water. If no nausea and/or vomiting occurs, water can be given. First aid consists of having the victim lie down in a cool place.

■ FROSTBITE ■

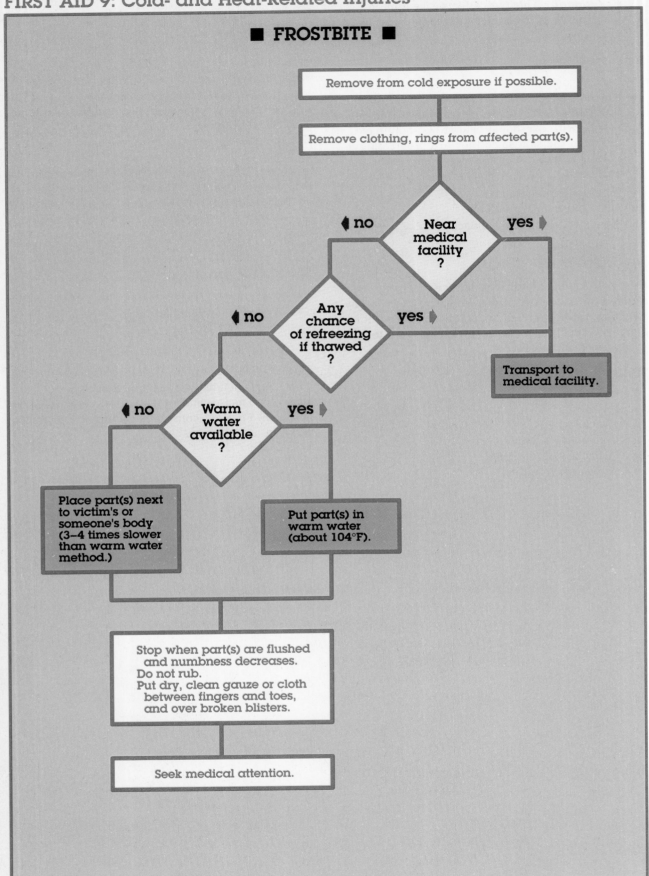

Remove from cold exposure if possible.

Remove clothing, rings from affected part(s).

Near medical facility?
- no
- yes → Transport to medical facility.

Any chance of refreezing if thawed?
- no
- yes → Transport to medical facility.

Warm water available?
- no → Place part(s) next to victim's or someone's body (3–4 times slower than warm water method.)
- yes → Put part(s) in warm water (about 104°F).

Stop when part(s) are flushed and numbness decreases.
Do not rub.
Put dry, clean gauze or cloth between fingers and toes, and over broken blisters.

Seek medical attention.

■ HYPOTHERMIA ■

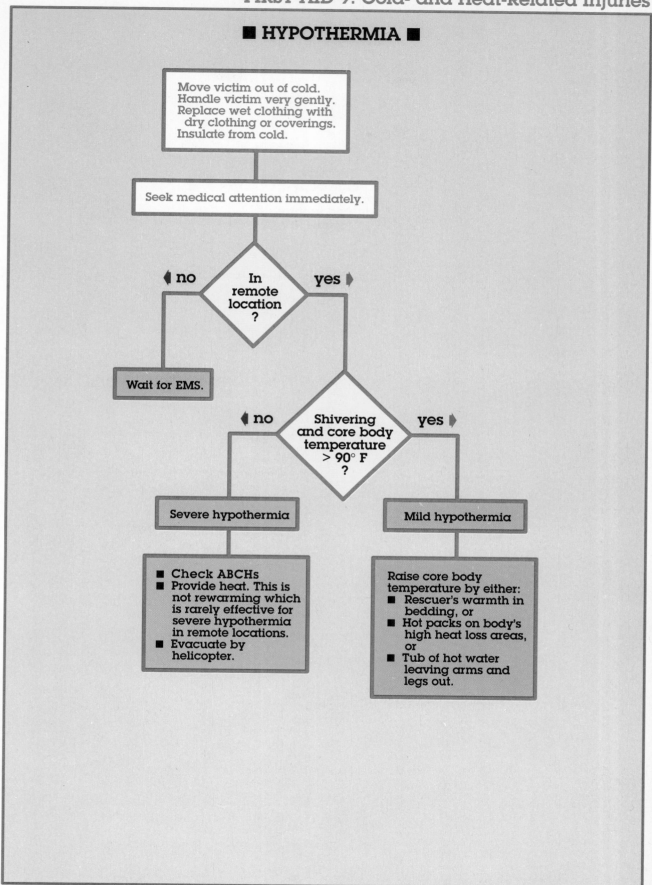

Move victim out of cold.
Handle victim very gently.
Replace wet clothing with
dry clothing or coverings.
Insulate from cold.

Seek medical attention immediately.

In remote location?

no — Wait for EMS.

yes

Shivering and core body temperature > 90° F ?

no — Severe hypothermia

- Check ABCHs
- Provide heat. This is not rewarming which is rarely effective for severe hypothermia in remote locations.
- Evacuate by helicopter.

yes — Mild hypothermia

Raise core body temperature by either:
- Rescuer's warmth in bedding, or
- Hot packs on body's high heat loss areas, or
- Tub of hot water leaving arms and legs out.

■ HEAT-RELATED EMERGENCIES ■

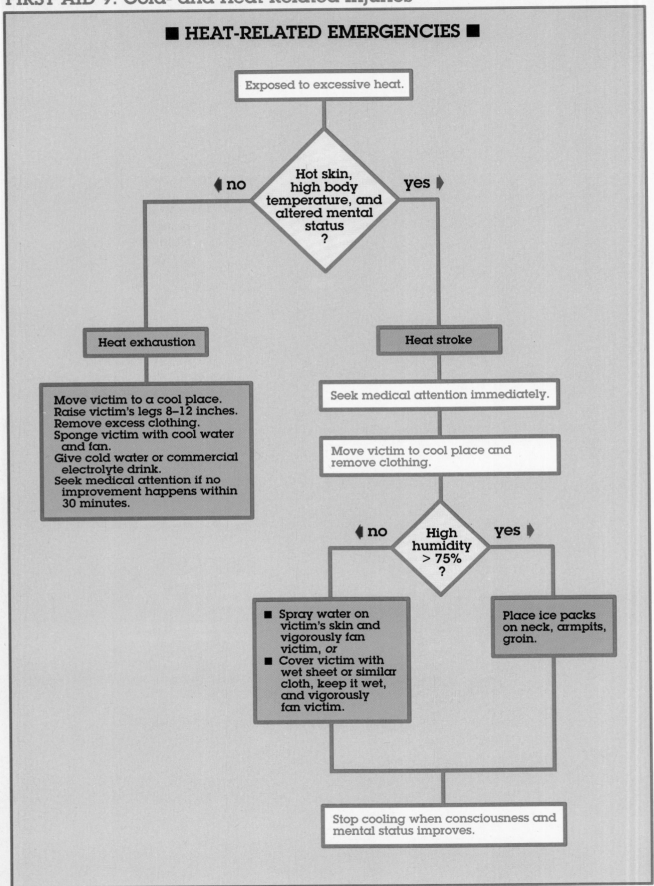

Exposed to excessive heat.

Hot skin, high body temperature, and altered mental status?

no → Heat exhaustion

Move victim to a cool place.
Raise victim's legs 8–12 inches.
Remove excess clothing.
Sponge victim with cool water and fan.
Give cold water or commercial electrolyte drink.
Seek medical attention if no improvement happens within 30 minutes.

yes → Heat stroke

Seek medical attention immediately.

Move victim to cool place and remove clothing.

High humidity > 75%?

no →
■ Spray water on victim's skin and vigorously fan victim, or
■ Cover victim with wet sheet or similar cloth, keep it wet, and vigorously fan victim.

yes →
Place ice packs on neck, armpits, groin.

Stop cooling when consciousness and mental status improves.

10

Bone, Joint, and Muscle Injuries*

Fractures

The terms **fracture** and **broken bone** have the same meaning—a break or crack in a bone. Fractures are classified as being **open** (when the skin is broken and bleeds externally) or **closed** (when the skin has not been broken).

Fracture Classification

- *Open (compound) fracture.* The overlaying skin has been damaged or broken. The wound can be produced either by the bone protruding through the skin or by a direct blow cutting the skin at the time of the fracture. The bone may not always be seen in the wound. Any broken bone which is covered by damaged skin is classified as an open fracture.
- *Closed (simple) fracture.* The skin has not been broken and no wound exists anywhere near the fracture site.

Open fractures are more serious than closed fractures because of greater blood loss and greater chance of infection.

Signs and Symptoms

- *Swelling.* Caused by bleeding; it occurs rapidly after a fracture.
- *Deformity.* This is not always obvious. Compare the injured with the uninjured opposite part when checking for deformity.
- *Pain and tenderness.* Commonly found only at the injury site. The victim will usually be able to point to the site of the pain. A useful procedure for detecting fractures is to gently feel along the bones; complaints about pain or tenderness serve as a reliable sign of a fracture.
- *Loss of use.* (Inability to use the injured part ("guarding"). Because motion produces pain, the victim will refuse to use it. However, sometimes the victim is able to move the limb with little or no pain.
- *Grating sensation.* Do *not* move the injured limb in an attempt to see if a grating sensation

Source: Based upon American Academy of Orthopaedic Surgeons protocols.

(called **crepitus**) can be felt and even sometimes heard when the broken bone ends rub together.

- *History of the injury.* suspect a fracture whenever severe accidents (e.g., motor-vehicle accidents and falls) happen. The victim may have heard or felt the bone snap.

Spinal Injuries

The spine is a column of vertebrae stacked one on the next from the skull's base to the tail bone. It encloses the spinal cord, which consists of long tracts of nerves that join the brain with all body organs and parts. It protects the spinal nerves.

If a broken spinal column pinches spinal nerves, paralysis can result. All unconscious victims should be treated as though they had spinal injuries. All conscious victims sustaining injuries from falls, diving accidents, auto accidents, or cave-in should be carefully checked for spine injuries before moving them.

A mistake in handling a spinal injured victim could mean a lifetime in a wheelchair or bed for the victim.

Signs and Symptoms

- Possible spinal injury in all severe accidents (e.g., motor-vehicle, falls, dives into water)
- Head injuries (They serve as a clue, since the head may have been snapped suddenly in one or more directions, endangering the spine. About 15% to 20% of head-injured victims also have neck and spinal cord injuries.)
- Painful movement of arms and/or legs
- Numbness, tingling, weakness, or burning sensation in arms or legs
- Loss of bowel or bladder control
- Paralysis to arms and/or legs
- Deformity (odd angle of the victim's head and neck)

Ask the conscious victim the following questions:

- *Is there pain?* Neck injuries (cervical) radiate pain to the arms; upper back injuries (thoracic) radiate pain around the ribs and into the chest; lower back injuries (lumbar) usually radiate pain down the legs. Often the victim describes the pain as "electric."

- **Can you move your feet?** Ask the victim to move his or her foot against your hand. If the victim cannot perform this movement or if the movement is extremely weak against your hand, the victim may have injured the cord.
- **Can you move your fingers?** Moving the fingers is a sign that nerve pathways are intact. Ask the victim to grip your hand. A strong grip indicates that a spinal cord injury is unlikely.

For an unconscious victim:

- Look for cuts, bruises, and deformities.
- Test responses by pinching the victim's hands (either palm or back) and feet (sole or top of the bare foot). No reaction could mean possible spinal cord damage.
- Ask others about what happened.

If not sure about a possible spinal injury, assume that the victim has one until proven otherwise.

Muscle Injuries

Though muscle injuries pose no real emergency, first aiders have ample opportunities to care for them.

Muscle Strains

A muscle strain, also known as muscle pull, occurs when the muscle is stretched beyond its normal range of motion, resulting in a muscle fiber tear. A range of severity exists.

Signs and Symptoms

- A sharp pain immediately after the injury
- Extreme tenderness when area is felt
- Disfigurement (indentation, cavity, or bump)
- Severe weakness and loss of function of the injured part
- The sound of a snap when the tissue is torn

Muscle Contusions

Muscle contusions result from a blow to a muscle. This injury is also known as a bruise.

Muscle Cramps

Muscles can go into an uncontrolled spasm and contraction, resulting in severe pain and a restriction or loss of movement. Some experts believe that diet or fluid loss explains muscle cramping. Nevertheless, many different things can cause muscle cramps; no one knows all the causes.

Cryotherapy

Ice is one of the most versatile treatments available for injuries. This form of treatment, called **cryotherapy,** uses ice or other cold applications for muscle strains, bruises, joint sprains, insect stings, and minor burns.

Reducing tissue temperature constricts blood vessels (helps by controlling bleeding), and reduces pain.

Forms of Ice Therapy

- **Ice massage.** Rubbing ice cubes in a circular motion on the affected area for 7 to 10 minutes on regions with little fat (e.g., elbow) and about 20 minutes in areas with more fat (e.g., leg muscles) is recommended.
- **Ice bags.** Apply a bag full of crushed ice or an ice cube to the affected area for 10 to 30 minutes. This method penetrates and lasts longer than the ice massage.
- **Cold water immersion.** An ice slush (ice cubes or crushed ice added to a bucket of water) is useful for injuries to the hand, foot, or elbow. Allow the injured part to soak in the ice slush for 10 to 20 minutes.
- **Cold packs.** Sealed plastic pouches containing a refreezable gel are available commercially. These can get very cold, so it is important that the cold packs be wrapped in a towel and that they never be applied directly to the skin.
- **Chemical "snap packs."** These sealed pouches resemble cold packs but contain two chemical envelopes that, when squeezed, mix the chemicals. A chemical reaction produces a cooling effect. Though they don't cool as well as other methods, snap packs are convenient.

Precautions include *NOT* exposing the skin to cold too long, which can result in frostbite. Those with any form of cold allergy, Raynaud's phenomenon, or abnormal sensitivity to cold should avoid cryotherapy.

Other tips when using ice or other forms of cryotherapy include the following:

- Apply ice or cold immediately after an injury.
- Raise the injured area above heart level.
- Apply ice or cold for no more than 30 minutes at a time. Repeat two to four times a day until fully recovered.

■ FRACTURES ■

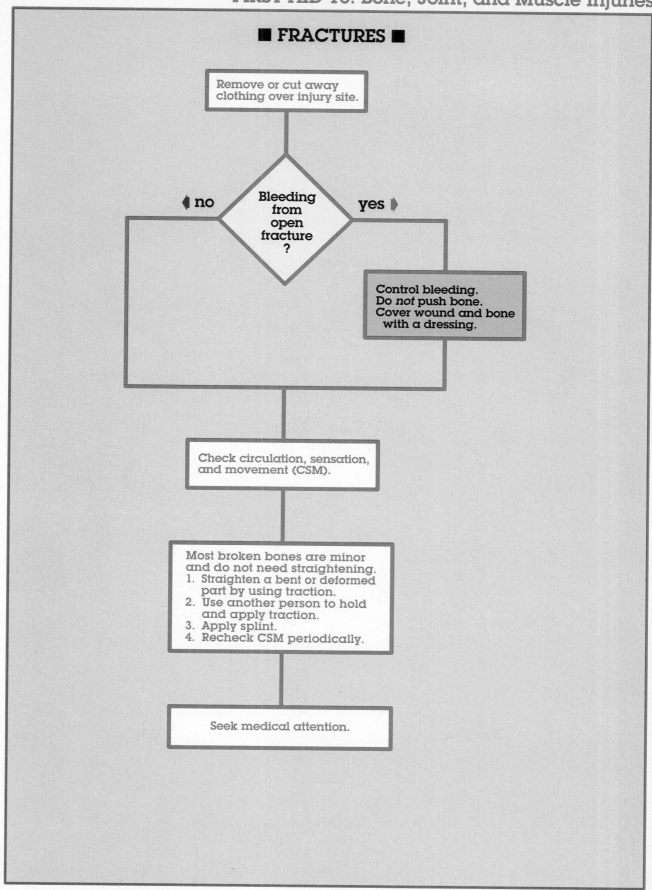

Remove or cut away clothing over injury site.

Bleeding from open fracture?

◀ no   yes ▶

Control bleeding.
Do *not* push bone.
Cover wound and bone with a dressing.

Check circulation, sensation, and movement (CSM).

Most broken bones are minor and do not need straightening.
1. Straighten a bent or deformed part by using traction.
2. Use another person to hold and apply traction.
3. Apply splint.
4. Recheck CSM periodically.

Seek medical attention.

■ SPINAL INJURIES ■

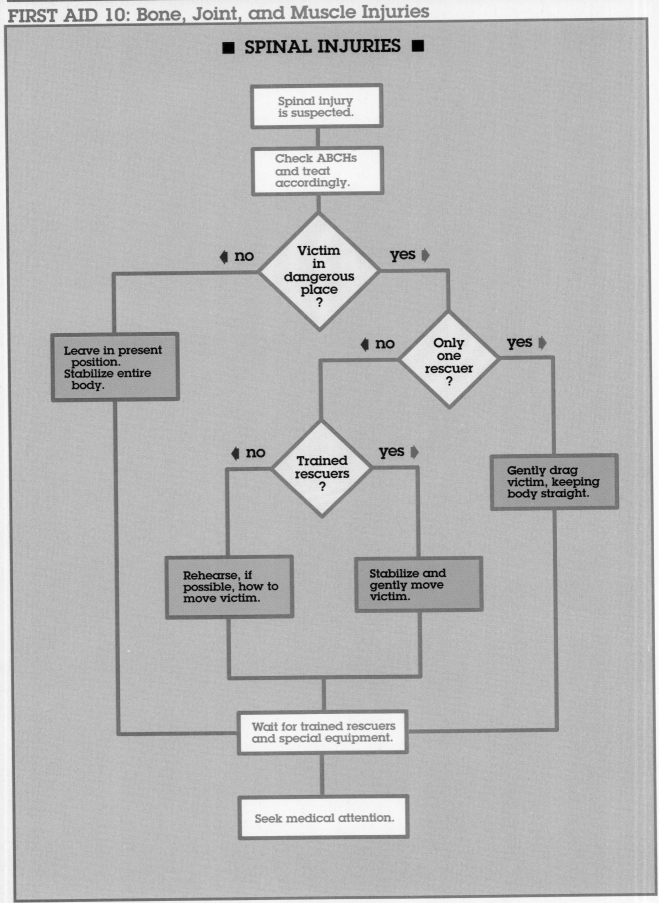

Spinal injury is suspected.

Check ABCHs and treat accordingly.

Victim in dangerous place ?

no → Leave in present position. Stabilize entire body.

yes → Only one rescuer ?

yes → Gently drag victim, keeping body straight.

no → Trained rescuers ?

no → Rehearse, if possible, how to move victim.

yes → Stabilize and gently move victim.

Wait for trained rescuers and special equipment.

Seek medical attention.

■ MUSCLE INJURIES ■

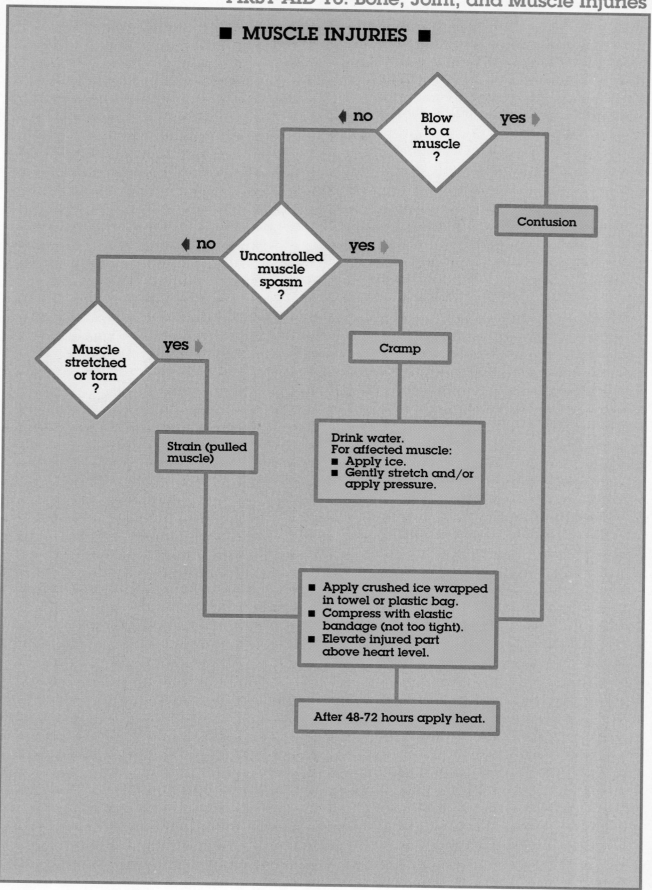

◀ **no** — **Blow to a muscle ?** — **yes** ▶

Contusion

◀ **no** — **Uncontrolled muscle spasm ?** — **yes** ▶

Muscle stretched or torn ? — **yes** ▶

Cramp

Strain (pulled muscle)

Drink water.
For affected muscle:
■ Apply ice.
■ Gently stretch and/or apply pressure.

■ Apply crushed ice wrapped in towel or plastic bag.
■ Compress with elastic bandage (not too tight).
■ Elevate injured part above heart level.

After 48-72 hours apply heat.

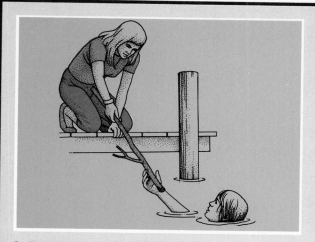

1. Reach the person from shore.

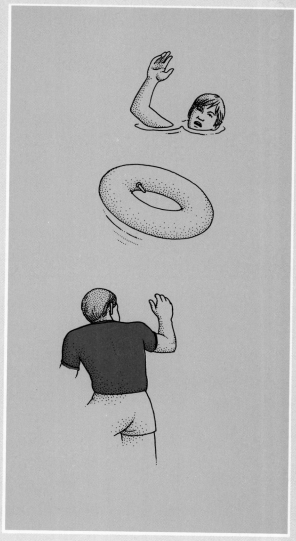

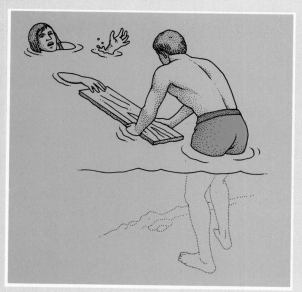

2. If you cannot reach the person from shore, wade closer.

3. If an object that floats is available, throw it to the person.

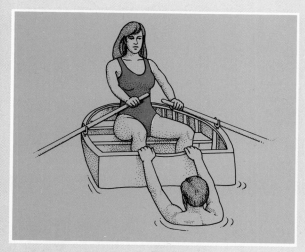

4. Use a boat if one is available.

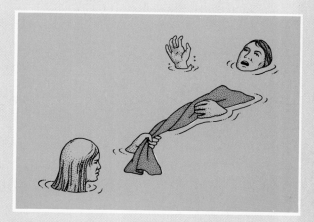

5. If you must swim to the person, use a towel or board for him or her to hold onto. Do not let the person grab you.

Quick Emergency Index